DRUGS & CONSEQUENCES

THE TRUTH ABOUT
BARBITURATES

JUDY MONROE PETERSON

Rosen
PUBLISHING

Published in 2014 by The Rosen Publishing Group, Inc.
29 East 21st Street, New York, NY 10010

Library of Congress Cataloging-in-Publication Data

Peterson, Judy Monroe.
The truth about barbiturates/Judy Monroe Peterson.—First edition.
    pages cm.—(Drugs & consequences)
Includes bibliographical references and index.
ISBN 978-1-4777-1896-4 (library binding)
1. Barbiturates—Juvenile literature. 2. Drug abuse—Juvenile literature.
I. Title.
RM325.P48 2014
615.7'821—dc23
                                                                2013013556

Manufactured in the United States of America

CPSIA Compliance Information: Batch #W14YA: For further information, contact Rosen Publishing, New York, New York, at 1-800-237-9932.

CONTENTS

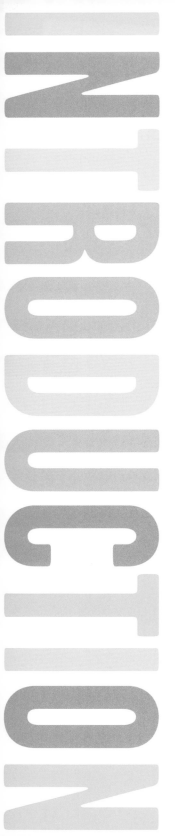

INTRODUCTION

Barbiturates are medically useful, man-made depressants. They slow down the activity of the central nervous system, which produces an array of effects from mild sedation to coma. Barbiturates, however, are widely misused. People intentionally take these substances to change how they think or feel when there is not a medical purpose to do so. Barbiturates have many street names, including "barbs," "block busters," "sleepers," and "downers."

Abuse of barbiturates and other prescription drugs is a serious problem in the United States, and it is the fastest-growing drug abuse trend among American teens. Every year, the National Institute on Drug Abuse (NIDA) conducts the Monitoring the Future survey to measure drug use among high school seniors. The data for 2011 shows that 14.8 percent of high school seniors had taken a prescription drug for nonmedical reasons in the past year. One category of misused prescription drugs is sedatives, which, in many cases, are barbiturates. Sedatives are depressants, or downers, that slow down the body and mind, causing people to feel relaxed and sleepy. Approximately 4.5 percent of surveyed teens reported nonmedical use of sedatives in 2011.

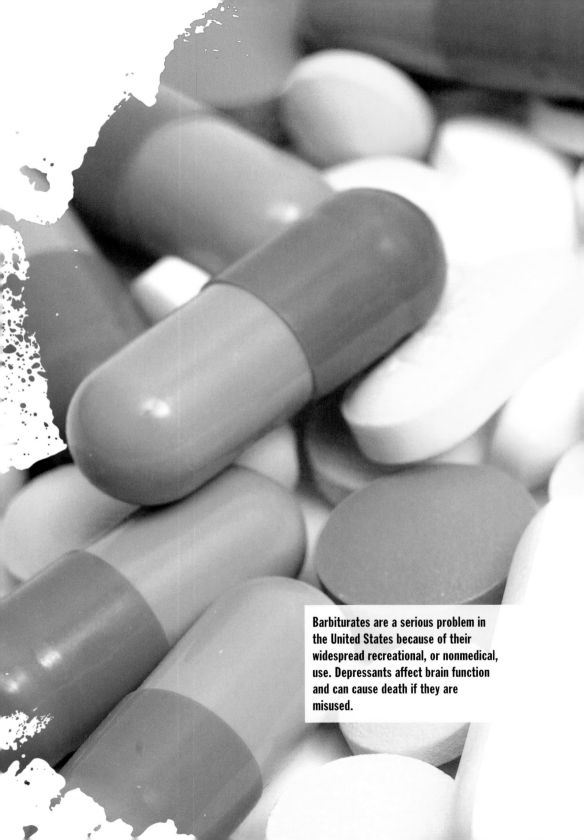

Barbiturates are a serious problem in the United States because of their widespread recreational, or nonmedical, use. Depressants affect brain function and can cause death if they are misused.

The Substance Abuse and Mental Health Services Administration (SAMHSA) is another federal agency that asks people about their drug use each year in the National Survey on Drug Use and Health. According to the 2011 survey results, 1.7 percent of young adults age eighteen to twenty-five used prescription drugs without a medical purpose. An estimated 2.4 million Americans used prescription drugs nonmedically for the first time in 2011. This number averages to about 2,200 initiates per day, of which one-third were twelve to seventeen years old.

Only physicians can prescribe barbiturates, which are generally safe when used properly. If barbiturates are mis-used, abusers can quickly develop a tolerance and need to take more of the drugs to achieve the original effects. Barbiturates are highly addictive. It can be difficult to stop once people start taking them. With higher doses, the chance of taking too much of the substances greatly increases, which can lead to coma or even death. Once addicted, it is hazardous to suddenly stop taking barbiturates because the substances affect the body's central nervous system, causing anxiety, insomnia, loss of appetite, muscle tremors, delirium, or seizures. Teens may not know that bar-biturates are extremely dangerous when they are combined with alcoholic beverages, such as beer, wine, or drinks con-taining rum, whiskey, or vodka. Both barbiturates and alcohol are central nervous system depressants, and the risk of overdosing is very high when they are taken together.

People who misuse barbiturates do not plan to develop an addiction. They take the drugs to experience specific mental and physical effects. Abusing these drugs, however, can result in addiction, permanent mental and physical harm, or even deadly reactions. In addition to affecting the abusers, drug use can affect family members, friends, and society. For instance, teens could cause a drug-related accident if they drive when feeling drowsy while using barbiturates. Knowing the facts about barbiturate abuse can help teens decide if taking these drugs is worth the risks. That decision is best made when people know what effects the substances have on their health and safety.

1

The Use of
Barbiturates Today

S ince the early 1900s, barbiturates have been important
   drugs in the treatment of an array of medical conditions. Their medical use declined, though, as other less
   addictive drugs began to replace them. Barbiturates
are not found in nature. Instead, they are manufactured in
chemical factories by pharmaceutical companies.

While working on his doctorate degree in Berlin, Germany, Adolf von Baeyer studied barbituric acid, which led to the manufacturing of barbiturates. He became a professor at the University of Munich in 1873, and in 1905, he won the Nobel Prize in Chemistry.

Discovery of Barbiturates

Adolf von Baeyer, a German scientist, discovered barbiturates in 1864 in his laboratory. He derived the substances from barbituric acid, an odorless, white powder that dissolves in water. At first, no one knew what to do with the

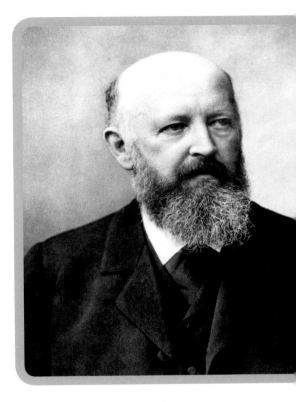

new drug. Then physicians began to learn that they could use it for various medical purposes, such as helping people fall asleep. Barbital was introduced as the first barbiturate in 1903 and was prescribed to treat anxiety disorders. The second one, phenobarbital, began selling in 1912 and soon became readily available by prescription. This substance was used to treat people who had epilepsy, a medical condition causing seizures. Phenobarbital helped control the number of seizures a person experienced. In addition to treating various medical conditions, barbiturates were given to people before surgery.

The drugs sedated the body, causing patients to feel no pain during an operation.

For about fifty years, barbiturates seemed almost like wonder drugs. Doctors thought that they were safe and effective and prescribed them for many health conditions. Over time, scientists created about 2,500 types of barbiturates from Baeyer's original formula, although most are based on the same basic chemical method. By the 1960s, people were reporting serious negative effects of the substances. Physicians discovered that people taking a barbiturate regularly over time usually developed a tolerance, meaning that they needed more and more of the drug to get the original effects. This increase in dosage led to a greater risk of overdosing. Another serious problem surfaced: barbiturates were found to be highly addictive.

Although these medicines remained effective, doctors began reducing their use because of the high risk for abuse. They began prescribing another class of depressants, benzodiazepines, to help people sleep or reduce their number of seizures. Like barbiturates, they are effective, but they have fewer side effects. Both types of medications are in use today, and both are available through a medical doctor's prescription.

Classes and Forms of Barbiturates

Most barbiturates are sorted into one of three categories according to how fast they work and how long they affect the body. The groups are short-acting, intermediate-acting,

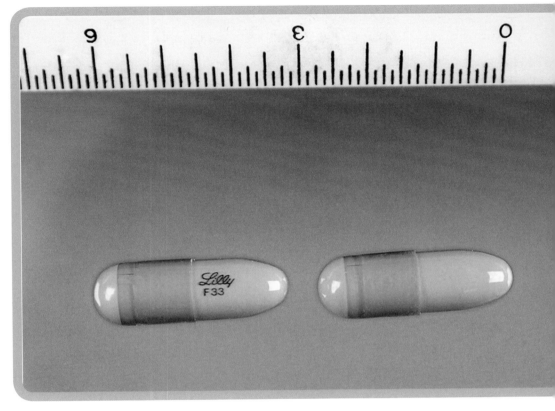

Amobarbital is a type of barbiturate that must be prescribed by a doctor and is used in the treatment of severe sleeping disorders. People feel drowsy after taking this medication, which helps them fall asleep at night.

and long-lasting. Short-acting barbiturates include pentobarbital and secobarbital. Their effects can remain in the body from three to four hours. Intermediates like amobarbital, aprobarbital, and butabarbital can continue to last six to eight hours. People who need to take a barbiturate regularly may use a long-lasting type, such as mephobarbital, phenobarbital, or primidone.

Another category of barbiturates is used as general anesthetics. Thiopental and methohexital are part of this group. The drugs are injected into a vein to quickly put someone to sleep, especially during emergency surgery. The effects start working immediately, usually within a minute. The person typically sleeps for less than thirty minutes. Doctors can keep giving doses of the drug during surgery until they want the patient to wake up and start to recover.

Sometimes physicians prescribe a group of barbiturates called combination analgesics for pain relief. These tablets or capsules are made up of a barbiturate and other drugs, such as caffeine, aspirin, or acetaminophen. Like other types of barbiturates, these combination drugs are available by prescription only.

Barbiturates are available in different forms. Depending on the medical needs of the patient, the drug may be taken by

DIFFERENCES BETWEEN SAFE AND UNSAFE DOSES

Barbiturate doses have a very small window between a safe dose and a lethal, or deadly, dose. People usually require just a tiny dose of the drug for treatment. Everyone reacts differently to a drug, based on his or her age, gender, weight, medical condition, dose of the drug, and how it is taken, such as a tablet or an injection. Doctors must carefully monitor their patients to determine the effects of the drug when they set, increase, or decrease the dose.

mouth, injected into a muscle or vein, or inserted as a capsule into the rectum. When injected into a vein, the substance goes directly into the bloodstream. Forms that are meant to be swallowed include tablets and capsules.

Current Medical Uses

Today, about twenty-five different barbiturates are in medical use in the United States. The drugs may not always be a doctor's first choice for treatment because of their risky effects, but they are still prescribed in some situations. For example, someone who is not helped by newer sedatives may be treated with barbiturates. Sometimes the substances work well when they are combined with a newer drug. Barbiturates are a physician's first choice for preventing seizures in infants. They are considered the most effective drug if the seizures are not deemed to be epilepsy. Infants usually outgrow their seizures and do not require barbiturates as a long-term treatment.

Another use of barbiturates is to treat a life-threatening seizure that can continue for minutes or hours. Most seizures last only a few seconds, but longer seizures can result in major damage to the body's organs and muscles. If people have this condition, they must go to a hospital immediately. There, the doctor will inject newer medications first. If these drugs fail, pentobarbital or secobarbital may be the next choice.

Sometimes veterinarians use barbiturates for treating seizures in dogs and other pets. The most commonly used drug

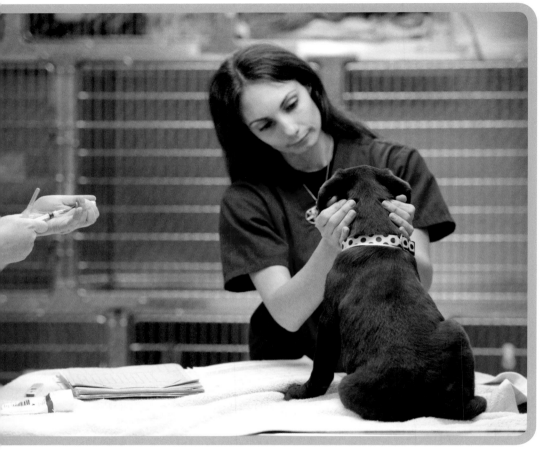

Phenobarbital can help control epilepsy in dogs and cats. It may also be used to treat seizures in horses if other types of drugs, such as benzodiazepines, are not effective.

for this condition is phenobarbital, which helps prevent seizures. The drug is given if the pet has more than one seizure every one or two months. As young pets grow into adults, they may stop having seizures naturally.

Prescription Drug Abuse

Although barbiturates are not prescribed as much today as in the past, they are still widely manufactured, sold, and used illegally. Street names for barbiturates are often based on how the colorful drugs look. Besides "barbs" and "block busters," these capsules and tablets are known as "Christmas trees," "goof balls," "phennies," "stumblers," and "tootsies." Other names are "rainbows," "pinks," "reds," "red devils," "reds and blues," "blue bombers," "blue devils," "blues," "yellows," "yellow jackets," and "purple hearts."

Abusers prefer the short-acting and intermediate barbiturates such as Amytal and Seconal. The short-acting drugs are usually more quickly addictive than the long-acting drugs. Teens report that they have easy access to these drugs at home because a family member is taking the medication and storing it in a bathroom medicine cabinet, drawer, or cupboard.

Most people typically swallow a barbiturate tablet or capsule or inject the liquid form of the drug. However, the drug is ordinarily taken by mouth. People tend to abuse barbiturates to reduce anxiety, decrease inhibitions, and treat the unwanted effects of other drugs that they have abused, such as cocaine, caffeine, or other stimulants. Unlike depressants, stimulants speed up the functions of the body and make people feel peppy. Barbiturates can be exceedingly dangerous if they are misused. Overdoses can lead to death. The National Institutes

of Health estimates that one out of ten people who experience a barbiturate overdose or mixture overdose will die,
usually from heart failure or lung problems.

The Law

Federal and state laws control prescription drugs, which regu-
late how the medications can be prescribed, sold, and used.
Prescription drugs can be obtained and used legally when prescribed by a physician. Some prescription drugs have high abuse
potential when they are taken in greater amounts than prescribed or when they are used by people for whom they are
not prescribed. The U.S. Drug Enforcement Agency (DEA) in
the Department of Justice regulates these drugs under the
Controlled Substances Act. Barbiturates and other controlled
substances are placed into one of five schedule categories

REGULATING DRUGS IN THE UNITED STATES

The U.S. Food and Drug Administration (FDA) serves as a consumer
watchdog for the thousands of prescription medications for sale. All
prescription medicines are regulated for safety and effectiveness. Before
a new product can be sold, the FDA extensively reviews the studies
conducted by the manufacturer. After an approved medication is on the
market, the FDA oversees the manufacturing, labeling, and advertising
of the medicine to monitor its safety.

based on findings such as the accepted medical use, the abuse potential, and the chance of addiction.

Drugs such as heroin and LSD have a significant abuse factor and no medical use. They are Schedule I drugs, meaning they cannot be prescribed by doctors. Barbiturates are Schedule II, III, and IV drugs because they have the potential to be abused. They require a prescription from a physician and are prescribed in a limited way. It is illegal to have an unauthorized possession or supply of barbiturates that is not prescribed. Schedule II substances cannot be refilled and have a greater chance of misuse than Schedule III and IV drugs. Schedule V drugs, such as aspirin, are available without a prescription and sold over the counter.

Physicians require a special license to get a DEA number for prescribing addictive substances such as barbiturates. They must be extremely careful when barbiturates are used by patients who have a history of drug abuse. By law, pharmacists are required to take extra steps when dispensing barbiturates and other controlled substances. For example, they need to keep detailed records of all controlled drugs for the FDA. Schedule II, III, and IV drugs must be kept in a locked area or secured at all times. Only pharmacy staff has access to this secured area.

CHAPTER 2

Dangers in

Society

S ometimes teens are faced with choices about drugs.
They have responsibilities and risks when it comes to
the use of any medication. The intentional misuse of
prescription drugs, such as barbiturates, includes giving
the substances to someone else or taking another person's
medication. Taking too much of a prescription drug or taking it
for a longer period of time than is prescribed are other ways
that people abuse drugs.

Why Drug Misuse Occurs

People use downers such as barbiturates for a variety of reasons. They think the drugs are a quick way to change their mood or help them relax. Some teens believe the drug's effects will be fun or provide a way to feel good, slow down, or decrease anxiety. Users may say that taking downers helps them escape from problems or cope with feelings of fear, depression, or pain. Teens may turn to them during times of transition, such as changing schools, moving, or

Some teens might be bullied at school but are afraid to tell someone about the problem. Instead, they may turn to sedatives, such as barbiturates, to feel less stressed.

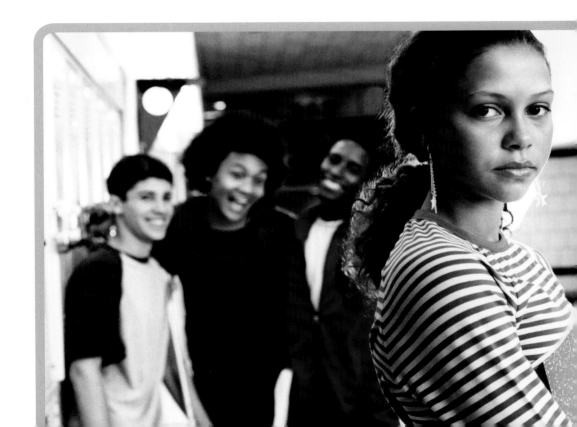

parental divorce. Others feel that they must perform well or even perfectly at school, work, or athletics and cope with this pressure by turning to barbiturates and other prescription medicines.

Some young people use drugs because they want to show that they are grown up, as a way to rebel against their parents, or to treat the unwanted effects of other drugs. A big reason, though, is that teens are bored or curious. Sometimes narcotic addicts substitute barbiturates for heroin if their supplies are cut.

Different factors influence a teen's decision to experiment with prescription drugs. One main reason is peer pressure, which can be a powerful force. Most teens want to fit in, be accepted, and have the approval of others. They may feel pressured to use drugs and do not know how to say no. Another situation that may influence teens is seeing a family member or friend misusing medications. Teens may lack a healthy role model, someone they admire and look up to. A role model can be a teacher, a coach, an athlete, other adults who do not abuse drugs, an older sibling, or someone in the media.

Teens may see drug misuse through the media, including ads, movies, and videos on TV and the Internet. Such messages can make drugs seem attractive and common. Sometimes the messages are accepted without much thought about the effects of the media's advertising. Teens may think the level of drug abuse is much more common than it really is.

Acquiring Barbiturates and Other Prescription Drugs

Barbiturate and other prescription drug abuse is a growing trend among teens. These drugs may be easy to get if medications are prescribed for one or more family members. The medicines are often stored unsecured in the bathroom or on a bedroom nightstand.

Friends or relatives may be another source of barbiturates and other prescription drugs. They can sell, share, or exchange with others who have prescription drugs at school. Teens might take

Taking barbiturates can temporarily mask feelings of sadness or low self-esteem, but over time barbiturates often increase anxiety or depression, which can end in death from overdosing or suicide.

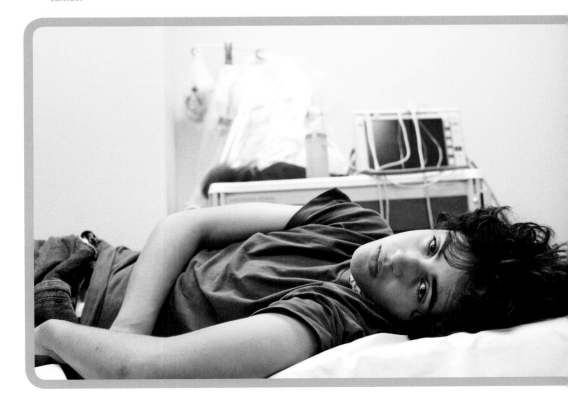

barbiturates at pharming parties when parents are out or in other social situations. For admittance to a pharming party, people bring prescription drugs, which are poured into a bowl and then mixed. Then they take turns swallowing one or more of the drugs. Some pharming parties are get-togethers for teens to barter for their favorite prescription drugs. Pharming is extremely dangerous because teens often do not know what drugs or how much they have swallowed. Taking a variety of medications at the same time can result in serious reactions, such as difficulty breathing or a rapid drop in heart rate. Teens may need to go to the emergency room for immediate treatment to avoid death.

Hardcore users take prescription drugs regularly, even daily, and find various ways to get their supply. They may steal drugs from a pharmacy. Some go to several different doctors to keep their use unnoticed. This practice is known as doctor shopping, and it is illegal. Addicts usually visit several pharmacies and are careful not to drop by one too often. Pharmacies keep track of how often they can refill a prescription for insurance payments and to catch people who are trying to get large amounts of drugs. Sometimes people may lie to their doctor, saying that it is still difficult to sleep or the dose is wearing off and needs to be increased. Others may go to different emergency rooms in the area, faking symptoms or using false names to get a prescription.

Abusers may write fake prescriptions by stealing or forging the prescription pads that doctors use. They may also alter a legitimate prescription by increasing the amount on the prescription or the number of refills. Today, many prescription pads are designed to be difficult to copy to prevent people from improperly obtaining drugs. Physicians are also steadily increasing their use of electronic prescriptions for medications. This technology helps reduce the possibility of prescription forgeries.

Using Online Pharmacies

Pharmacies available on the Internet are growing in popularity because people can shop twenty-four hours a day. Some online pharmacies provide safe services. Legitimate pharmacies are licensed in the United States and have an actual telephone number and address. They require prescriptions and have a pharmacist onsite who is available for questions.

Sadly, the number of illegal online pharmacies is expanding. Teens can access these Web sites at any time and may receive offers of prescription drugs through e-mail spam or pop-ups. These vendors usually do not require prescriptions for purchasing their medications. The drugs they sell are often unregulated and may be counterfeit, impure, or expired. The medications might be the wrong dose strength, may be inappropriate for the person's weight, or don't provide dosage information or any warnings, such as side effects and drug interactions. In addition, people usually don't know if the prescriptions were stored and shipped under proper conditions, such as the need for refrigeration.

Taking unregulated drugs could cause teens to have no improvement in their medical condition or make it worse. Medicines may have unknown ingredients or slight variations

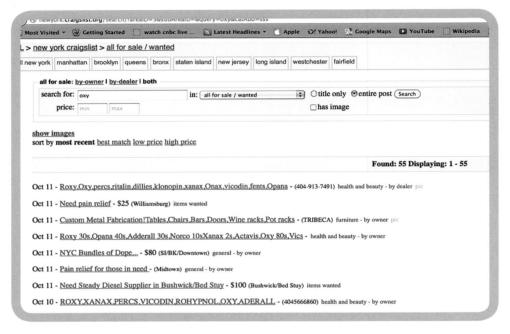

newyork.craigslist.org/search/raralD=5&subAealD=&query=oxy&catADD=sss

| Most Visited ▾ | Getting Started | watch cnbc live ... | Latest Headlines ▾ | Apple | Yahoo! | Google Maps | YouTube | Wikipedia |

L > new york craigslist > all for sale / wanted

| ll new york | manhattan | brooklyn | queens | bronx | staten island | new jersey | long island | westchester | fairfield |

all for sale: by-owner I by-dealer I both

search for: oxy   in: all for sale / wanted   ○ title only ● entire post (Search)

price: min   max   ☐ has image

show images
sort by **most recent** best match low price high price

Found: 55 Displaying: 1 - 55

Oct 11 - Roxy,Oxy,percs,ritalin,dillies,klonopin,xanax,Onax,vicodin,fents,Opana - (404-913-7491) health and beauty - by dealer pic

Oct 11 - Need pain relief - $25 (Williamsburg) items wanted

Oct 11 - Custom Metal Fabrication!Tables,Chairs,Bars,Doors,Wine racks,Pot racks - (TRIBECA) furniture - by owner pic

Oct 11 - Roxy 30s,Opana 40s,Adderall 30s,Norco 10sXanax 2s,Actavis,Oxy 80s,Vics - health and beauty - by owner

Oct 11 - NYC Bundles of Dope... - $80 (SI/BK/Downtown) general - by owner

Oct 11 - Pain relief for those in need - (Midtown) general - by owner

Oct 11 - Need Steady Diesel Supplier in Bushwick/Bed Stuy - $100 (Bushwick/Bed Stuy) items wanted

Oct 10 - ROXY,XANAX,PERCS,VICODIN,ROHYPNOL,OXY,ADERALL - (4045666860) health and beauty - by owner

People sometimes steal prescription drugs that are readily available at home and sell them illegally on the Internet. When police spot the ads, they arrest these drug dealers.

and could cause harmful effects. A drug's effects may be multiplied beyond what is intended, and that could be deadly. For example, people have died after taking barbiturates and alcohol together. Both are depressants and can shut down respiration and other vital functions of the body.

Risks

Barbiturate and other prescription drug misuse is a high-risk behavior. It can be a factor with teens who have been involved in crime, suicide, traffic accidents, and hospital admissions.

FAKE INTERNET PHARMACIES

Illegal online pharmacies can often be spotted because they sell drugs at cheap prices, ship worldwide, or allow anyone to buy medications without a prescription. In addition, they are not usually located or licensed in the United States. It is smart to buy only from an American pharmacy licensed with its state board of pharmacy. People can go to the Web site of the National Association of Boards of Pharmacy to see lists of recommended and not recommended online pharmacies. To report a suspicious Internet pharmacy site, call the DEA hotline at (877) 792-2873, or file a report at http://www.nabp.net/programs/accreditation/vet-vipps/report-a-site. The hotline is open around the clock, 365 days a year.

Prescription drug abuse may cause teens to have unprotected sex and increase their risk of unwanted pregnancy or exposure to sexually transmitted diseases such as herpes and the human immunodeficiency virus (HIV).

Possessing or using prescription drugs without a doctor's prescription is against the law. According to the DEA, giving or selling these drugs to someone else shows the intent to distribute. Breaking the law has consequences. Illegal distribution or the possession of prescribed medications often leads to fines, prison time, jail bond, and probation. It could also result in the loss of a driver's license, court-ordered drug treatment, and other penalties.

Additional serious consequences can result with prescription drug misuse. Teens may pay for accidents that occurred

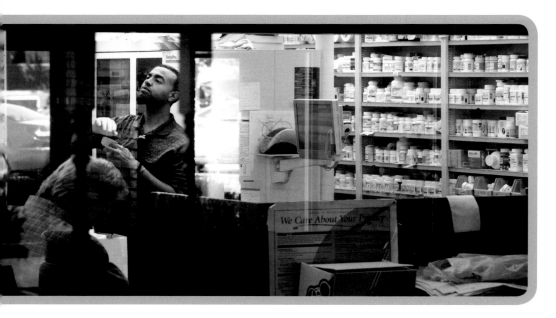

When the Drug Enforcement Administration (DEA) audited the records of medicines in this pharmacy, more than 100,000 prescription drugs were missing. As a result, the DEA seized all of the pharmacy's medications.

while they were under the influence of a drug. Some teens brag about their illegal drug use on social networking Web sites such as Facebook or Twitter. This information is available to future employers, college admissions offices, and others. Their drug misuse can ruin their chances of being accepted by the military or being hired for certain jobs. Being caught for substance abuse is easily accomplished with blood or urine tests.

MYTHS & FACTS

MYTH Prescription drugs are safer than illegal drugs, such as cocaine or heroin.

FACT Drugs prescribed by physicians are typically safe if they are taken exactly as prescribed and for the intended purpose. When they are abused, prescription drugs can be addictive and put abusers at risk for an overdose, especially when taken along with other drugs or alcohol.

MYTH It is normal for teens to experiment and misuse barbiturates and other prescription drugs.

FACT Experimenting with prescription drugs is not normal. Most teens don't misuse prescription drugs. Using them improperly can lead to abuse, which can become an addiction.

MYTH Bathroom cabinets or drawers are the best places to store barbiturates and other prescription drugs.

FACT Bathrooms may not be the best place to keep medications. All medicine should be placed in a locked container and stored in a safe place. It's a good idea to count medications and monitor their use to determine if someone is misusing them. Another safeguard is always to dispose of old or unused medications properly. People can contact their local government to determine if a drug take-back program is available in their area.

The **Impact** on the **Body** and **Mind**

W hen taken correctly, prescription drugs are extremely important for many people. Barbiturates are powerful depressant drugs and can be helpful when dealing with anxiety attacks, sleep disorders, and seizures. Medications can also be unsafe if they are abused. Only trained health professionals can predict the effects of a specific barbiturate and dose for a person. Each person reacts differently to an identical dose.

Short-Term Effects

The short-term effects that barbiturates have on the body depend on various factors, such as what drug and how much of that drug is swallowed, the person's size and gender, and whether or not other drugs are used. At first, people may feel calm, peaceful, or relaxed. Their inhibitions are lowered and may cause them to take even more of the drug. People can feel that they are escaping from the problems of their daily lives. Barbiturates and other depressants slow the work of the central nervous system and cause sleepiness. However, some users may feel euphoria, which is an exaggerated sense of well-being. Barbiturates depress normal brain function. Users may be tired, slur their speech, be unsteady when moving around, or have difficulty focusing their eyes. The effects typically last from six to seven hours but may produce a hangover effect.

After taking barbiturates and then sleeping, a hangover can occur the next day. This sick, uncomfortable state comes from the misuse of barbiturates or other depressants, such as alcohol. People may feel dizzy, shaky, irritable, or anxious. Some have an upset stomach, are sensitive to light and sound, or may have a headache or muscle aches and pain.

Similar to a hangover, short-term use of barbiturates temporarily dulls the brain and body. People may have problems with their memory and coordination. Their judgment becomes impaired and the speed of responses or action can be reduced.

Impaired judgment can cause poor performance in school, athletics, or work. In addition, teens may fall asleep when they are driving or handling power tools, which can lead to a serious accident. When users ingest barbiturates and alcohol at the same time, the body may try to reject the drugs by vomiting. If they are lying down and unable to get up, they could suffocate on their own vomit and die.

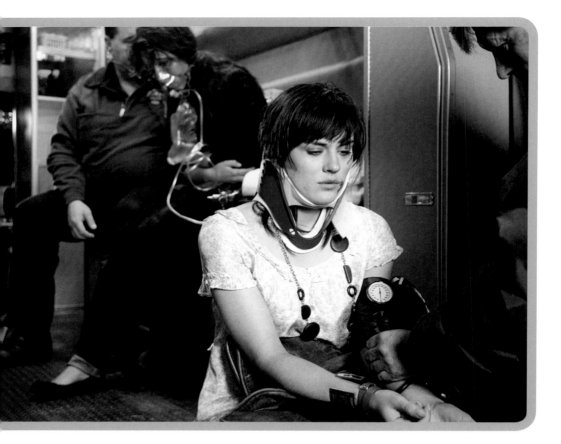

As depressants, barbiturates can cause sleepiness and affect judgment, coordination, and memory. For those who drive, barbiturate use can lead to a greater likelihood of having car accidents.

Long-Term Effects

People using barbiturates regularly may soon develop a tolerance. They need larger or more frequent doses to achieve the drug's original effects. Some teens may try to control their use of barbiturates, but they cannot. Instead, they grow increasingly dependent on the drug.

Dependence develops when a person starts to crave the barbiturate. Two types of dependence, physical and psychological, are both at work with barbiturates. Some teens have a chemical need for the substance. If drug use is reduced or stopped suddenly, very unpleasant withdrawal reactions, seizures, or other harmful consequences may result. Those teens with a psychological dependence think more barbiturates are needed to feel good or function

INJECTING BARBITURATES

Sometimes addicts inject a barbiturate-water mix into a vein or muscle. Taking barbiturates in this way is especially dangerous. Users do not know how much of the substance they are getting or what ingredients may be in the solution. They can introduce unknown drugs into the bloodstream, leading to serious damage to the veins or circulatory system. If people inject the drug into an artery by mistake, they may develop skin abscesses. The risk of gangrene greatly increases, too. Drug users frequently share dirty needles or syringes and can contract serious diseases, such as HIV, tetanus, hepatitis, or other infections.

normally. They may feel that normal life is too unbearable without the drugs. They continue to use barbiturates for their effects of relieving feelings of stress, loneliness, or anxiety. These people are addicted and need professional help to quit.

Some users combine drugs, such as barbiturates and alcohol, which can cause dependency on more than one kind of drug. They require more of the drugs and often have a difficult time quitting or cannot stop using the drugs. People need the drugs to stop violent shaking or to avoid feeling sick.

By now, users may have an addiction, or the physical and psychological dependence on a drug. Barbiturates are especially dangerous because an addiction can develop quickly—in about two weeks or less. People continue to take the substances despite the harmful consequences, and using barbiturates becomes their main goal in life. At this point, they may have suffered a major loss as a result of their addiction. Some teens get suspended from school, lose their job, or cause a traffic accident as a result of heavy drug use.

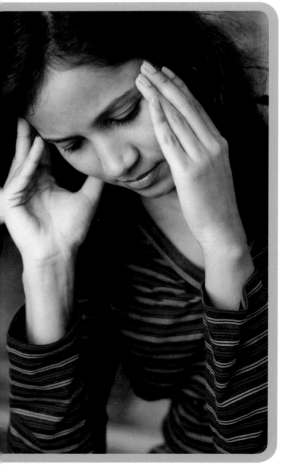

When teens abuse barbiturates regularly, their tolerance for the drugs' effects on mood develops faster than their tolerance for a lethal dose. Consequently, people run increasingly higher risks of accidentally killing themselves by overdosing.

Many people begin to feel physically and emotionally exhausted, which can lead to suicide.

As people take increasingly higher doses of a barbiturate, the risk of overdosing greatly rises. Long-term use of barbiturates can negatively affect learning abilities or damage the brain. Users don't feel refreshed after they sleep. Barbiturate abuse can harm essential organs, such as the heart, making users

ADDICTION: A BRAIN DISEASE

Addiction to barbiturates is a brain disease because the drugs change the structure of the brain and how it works on the central nervous system, or CNS. The CNS controls nearly everything that keeps a body alive, such as heart rate, blood flow, breathing, digestion, reflexes, memory, sleeping, thoughts, and more. The brain operates by receiving information from the senses, deciding how the body should respond, and then sending instructions to trigger the actions. Scientists do not fully understand how barbiturates work inside the brain. The drugs may activate a necessary brain chemical known as gamma-aminobutyric acid (GABA). These chemical messengers tell different body functions to slow down.

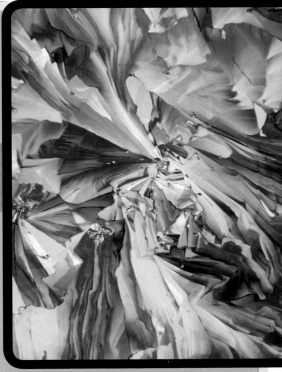

Glutamic acid crystals, as seen here through a special microscope, are naturally occurring in the brain. They are necessary for the formation of gamma-aminobutyric acid (GABA), an essential part of the central nervous system.

more susceptible to disease. As the heart becomes weaker, it decreases the pumping of blood rich in oxygen through the body. Judgment and coordination are gravely impaired. At extremely high doses, different body functions may begin to shut down. The digestive system may not be able to move food and liquids to the stomach and intestines for processing. Breathing becomes difficult because the respiratory system operates inefficiently. Death can be the end result.

Drug Interactions, Overdose, and Withdrawal

Barbiturates taken with a wide variety of other drugs can change how the liver processes them. The liver regulates the levels of most of the main chemicals in the body by clearing the blood of drugs and poisonous substances. The organ does this by absorbing substances, changing their chemical structure, and then filtering waste from the blood.

Serious drug interactions can occur when multiple medicines are taken together. Prescription and nonprescription depressants increase the depressive side effects of barbiturates. Common depressants include antihistamines, tranquilizers, and alcohol. Antihistamines are in prescription and nonprescription allergy and cold medications. Barbiturates used with other depressants increase the speed by which the liver processes and eliminates numerous drugs. As a result, many beneficial medications, such as corticosteroids for treating rheumatoid arthritis, are poorly processed and less effective.

A person can die from an overdose of barbiturates. An overdose is a strong reaction to taking a large amount of the drug alone or along with alcohol or other depressants, such as heroin, or OxyContin, a narcotic pain reliever. At the early stages of an overdose, people may become extremely disoriented and have very poor coordination and impaired thinking. They may try to fight people providing medical help. However, the drugs can quickly subdue a person's breathing to the point that a coma or respiratory arrest occurs.

If people abruptly stop using barbiturates, they may go through withdrawal. The body may react violently by vomiting, sweating, trembling, or having convulsions (abnormal muscle contractions). Seizures or bleeding in the brain can occur, and the circulatory system can be seriously weakened, leading to coma or death.

4

Identifying
Barbiturate
Abuse

B arbiturate misuse and abuse can cause grave problems for users. Using the drugs inappropriately even once can result in serious, negative reactions or possibly death. Regular abusers probably cannot fully partici-pate in society because of their physical and psychological problems. This absence can be damaging to family, friends, and other people. People can experience severe allergic reactions to a barbiturate, thus requiring immediate medical care. Permanent psychological and physical damage, including loss of the ability to learn, can also result.

Misusing barbiturates can cause teens to fall asleep at inappropriate times and perform poorly at school. Users then might strain personal relationships by asking friends to do their schoolwork.

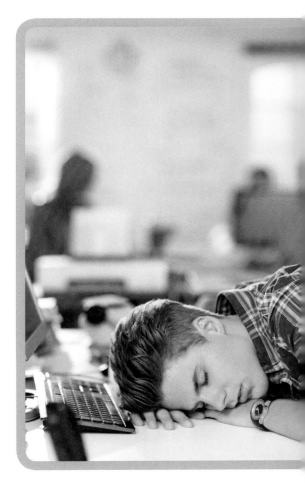

Why Look for a Drug Abuser?

Addicts frequently put great strain on their family and damage relationships. To keep their drug use a secret, they may take great pains to keep from being caught while using. They might lie and make up excuses for staying out late. As their own drug funds dwindle, some teens ask family members for loans but never repay their debt. They may steal money from parents or siblings, or sell a valuable household item to raise money for buying drugs. Abusers can become rude and intimidating toward their family and provide a bad example for younger siblings.

Users typically have many social issues. Teens may steal and lie to friends to get money for buying drugs. Their friends may feel hurt or angry and pull away. Abusers tend to withdraw from their friends and seek out those who also use and buy drugs. They have difficulty understanding how their negative actions affect friends and other people.

Drug abusers have an effect on society in many ways. To pay for their addiction, they may become involved in theft, prostitution, selling drugs, or stealing barbiturates from neighborhood homes or pharmacies. Such actions increase the crime rate in the United States. If teens have a job, they may have trouble doing their tasks, such as taking or filling orders at a restaurant or store. Conflicts with coworkers, criticism from a supervisor, falling asleep on the job, or causing injuries in the workplace occur more often. Workers abusing drugs perform less efficiently, make more mistakes, and damage property. The result is an increased risk of causing dangerous accidents. Such irresponsible behaviors often lead to being fired from the job.

The cost to society for drug abuse is staggering. People who overdose or engage in violent crime often need to go to emergency rooms, which increases health care costs for everyone. They may miss a lot of work, resulting in lost wages. Teens may have to take lower-paying jobs because of poor grades and higher dropout rates from schools. People commiting crimes under the influence of drugs may end up in court, increasing legal costs for the community. Finally, drug abuse can shorten the life span of addicts or waste years of their lives because they spend most of their time thinking about, getting, and using barbiturates. They may lose out on growing, learning, and enjoying life. Making close, personal friends becomes difficult or impossible.

Identifying a Drug Abuser

Drug addiction usually does not develop immediately. It is a more gradual process, although barbiturate addiction can occur quite quickly, in two weeks or less. Teens can watch for warning signs indicating someone they know has a drug problem. The negative changes may be different for each person.

Drug abusers can lose interest in friends, hobbies, athletics, or clubs. They may skip school, sleep too much, lose weight suddenly, or have low energy and difficulty making decisions, concentrating, or learning. Grades on report cards drop. Teens may perform badly in school, athletics, or work, or just stop showing up. Some people don't keep their body or clothes clean and are sick more often than in the past. Users may feel rebellious, angry, restless, or irritable, or think about death and suicide.

Family members and friends may see other signs of a drug dependency. Abusers become secretive and hide things, avoid eye contact, lock their bedroom door or dressers, and take drugs alone. If teens are absent from home, school, or work, they seldom provide an explanation. People might panic if their drug supply is low or runs out, rely on drugs to forget problems or relax, or deny that they have a problem.

Handling an Overdose

Getting help fast for someone who may have overdosed on barbiturates could mean the difference between life and death. If the person is extremely tired or has breathing difficulties, someone should immediately call a local emergency number, such as 911. The American Association of Poison Control Centers Help Line can be called from anywhere in the United States, at (800) 222-1222. Experts there provide instructions about an overdose. This free, confidential service is available twenty-four hours a day, seven days a week.

If no immediate emergency help is available, the person should be taken to the nearest hospital or medical facility. The name of the drug, the amount taken, and the time it was ingested is very helpful information for medical personnel. If available, it's a good idea to give the drug bottles or other containers to emergency staff.

Poison control centers are medical facilities where doctors, nurses, and pharmacists provide free and immediate treatment help over the telephone in cases involving the misuse of substances such as sedatives.

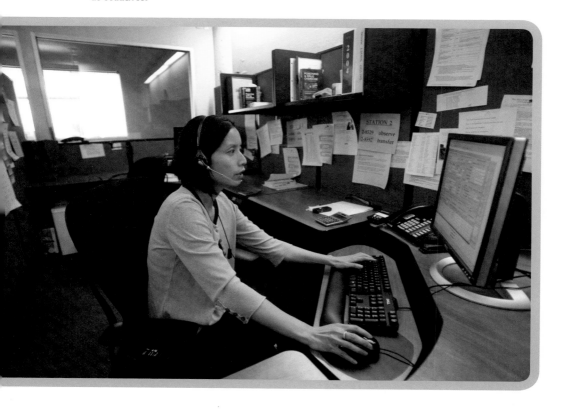

Until medical help arrives, it is important to check and monitor the overdosed person's airway, breathing, and pulse. Cardiopulmonary resuscitation (CPR) may be necessary. The person should be kept warm and calm and not be allowed to take more drugs. Some people may be in shock and are weak and pale, and have blue lips and fingernails and shallow breathing. The skin may feel clammy. Treating seizures requires first aid for convulsions.

Doctors can't provide a drug to help reverse the effects of barbiturate overdose. However, they may give the person activated charcoal. This substance helps absorb barbiturates,

BARBITURATES AND DRIVING

Abusing barbiturates impairs people's thinking and reacting, and it decreases their coordination, judgment, and reflexes. They may behave carelessly while driving. People who are abusing drugs are more likely than nonusers to cause or be in a traffic accident and injure or kill others. They may be arrested and charged with one or more crimes. Abusers may be required to take drug abuse education classes, which they must pay for. Their vehicle may be towed and stored, and to get it back, they must pay a fee. Sometimes parents pay bail bond fees for the release of their teen who is in prison. In addition, auto insurance companies increase their rates or cancel the policy. Then teens and their families must buy expensive, high-risk auto insurance. If they are found guilty of driving while they are on drugs, people can lose their license and must pay to get it returned. In addition, the crime will stay on their record.

keeping the drugs from moving to the stomach and intestines. If someone is in a coma or is not breathing well, a breathing tube is inserted in his or her throat. Over time, breathing can deepen and the person may come out of the coma. However, survival from an overdose is not guaranteed.

Drug Testing and the Law

Drug tests analyze what substances are in urine, blood, hair, saliva, or sweat. Blood and urine tests are the most common tests used to screen for drugs. A urine test costs the least and can detect drug use that has occurred within the past week. However, the test can be affected if teens do not use drugs for a period of time before the test. In other words, there is a limited window of detection time for a urine test. A blood test is the most costly, but it is the most accurate.

Random drug testing can occur at work, at school, and with school-sponsored athletics teams. Drug testing is used in hospital emergency rooms for suspected drug overdoses and when arrests for driving violations suggest that there has been drug abuse. If positive results occur, teens may be suspended from school or athletic groups. They probably can't apply for many jobs and might be fired from their current job or go to a mandatory treatment program.

Some parents use a home drug-testing program to determine if their teen is using drugs. The kits may come with a

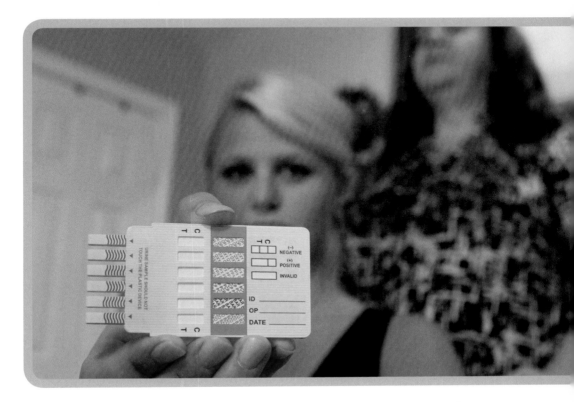

Parents who are concerned about their teens abusing prescription and other drugs may do drug testing at home. Drug testing kits, such as this one, can help parents monitor possible drug misuse.

thermometer for parents to check if the body temperature is the same as the sample urine. If the sample urine is cold, the teen used a sample from someone else. Using a temperature test makes it more difficult for teens to manipulate test results. People report that the kits are easy to use and produce a positive or negative test. If the test is positive, a laboratory must verify the results.

TEN

1. My parents have a history of drug abuse. Is this barbiturate safe for me to use?

2. How will I know if my barbiturate medication is working?

3. What should I do if side effects occur while taking barbiturates?

4. What substances or food should I avoid when using barbiturates?

5. How do I prevent developing dependence or addiction to barbiturates?

6. I have been taking too much of a barbiturate regularly. How can I stop this drug safely?

7. Is there a program or clinic that can help me stop using barbiturates?

8. What should I do if the current dose of my barbiturate prescription is not helping me?

9. Do you know anyone I can talk to who has been through barbiturate use and withdrawal?

10. How can I get tested to determine if I have any damage to my brain and body from abusing barbiturates?

CHAPTER 5

Building a
Healthy
Lifestyle

Taking the first step in getting help with barbiturate abuse requires teens to admit that they have a problem. Users may be in denial about their drug abuse, which prevents them from seeking help. Denial is when people refuse to admit how much of a drug they use or how frequently they use it. The second step toward recovery is to tell someone who can help you begin the treatment process. Teens may find that family and friends are willing to provide support throughout the process.

Getting Started

To get started, teens must decide to end their addiction to barbiturates. Asking for help is a difficult action for people in denial, but it is essential to overcoming substance abuse. Sometimes teens must get treatment when they have had many bad things happen to them because of their addiction, including getting a sexually transmitted disease or getting arrested. People might have to enter a drug treatment program because of the problems they caused while on substances. Teens may need to shop around to get professionals who best work with their personalities.

Some teens do not tell anyone about their barbiturate abuse. However, the first step in obtaining help for themselves is to tell someone who is trustworthy about their drug use.

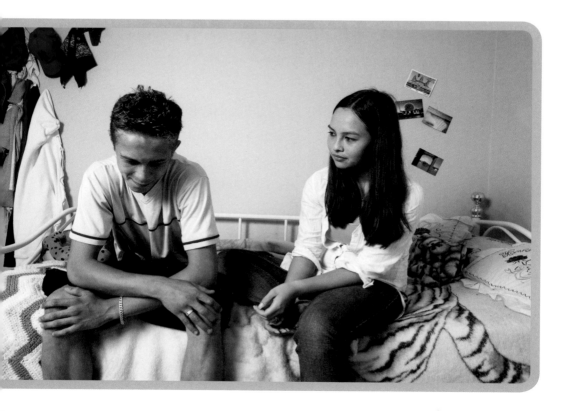

The most important part of getting help is that abusers tell someone they trust about their drug use. Before the discussion, people may find it useful to write down what they want to say and then memorize it. Teens may decide to talk with a parent, guardian, or parent of a friend. Other supportive family members can be an older sibling, aunt, or grandparent. Teens might turn to an understanding friend or family doctor to admit their drug use. School teachers, social workers, psychologists, guidance counselors, nurses, and coaches can provide support. They may be in touch with local substance abuse programs. Many places of worship provide drug programs. Religious leaders in the community, including priests, rabbis, pastors, ministers, or imams, can also help. Teens may decide to go to a local drop-in center or dependency unit, if one is available.

People may be more comfortable calling an anonymous hotline, where trained counselors listen and provide support. All information is confidential. The Internet or a local telephone book usually lists abuse hotlines in the community. Another option for teens is calling a national hotline. They don't need to provide any personal details to these hotlines. Counselors provide information about drug use and how to recover from drug abuse and addiction. They may recommend what to do next and supply contact information for local counselors, therapists, or programs. These people can help teens prepare what they might want to say to their parents when they admit to them that they have a drug problem.

Withdrawal

People must get barbiturates out of their body to begin dealing with their addiction. To do this, they need to stop taking the drug safely. It is highly recommended that this process is carried out under the guidance of doctors in a hospital or detoxification facility. Before teens go through withdrawal, physicians evaluate them physically and mentally. They order drug tests to determine what substances are present in the body. After the information is collected and evaluated, teens begin the withdrawal process. They are

THERAPY FOR TEENS AND THEIR FAMILY

Therapy sessions can be intense and difficult. Teens may want to meet with a few therapists before choosing one. People can ask about their training, certification, and experience, and what they can do to help. It is important to select a therapist who is respectful and gives hope that teens can feel better. Therapists talk about treatment and recovery choices that people have and what to do if something is not working for them. They might see individuals alone or the family as a whole. Family therapy helps build support between teens and their family members who may have difficulty relating to each other. These relationships may become especially difficult and upsetting during drug addiction. Therapy can help teens and family members work together to make positive and supportive changes in everyone's life.

given lower and lower doses of barbiturates while being closely monitored by a physician.

Withdrawal can take days or even weeks. The length of time depends on various factors, such as how large the final doses were and the dose strength. A person's size and physical condition also impact withdrawal. If this procedure is rushed, the consequences can be seizures and possibly death.

During this process, people may experience uncontrollable tremors affecting their entire body. Some lose their appetite, have an upset stomach, sweat a lot, or feel dizzy and anxious. Insomnia or vivid dreams and nightmares can occur. Their heart rate may be high, and breathing can be difficult. In some cases, people may have hallucinations (seeing and hearing things that are not there).

Treatment

After completing barbiturate withdrawal, teens usually require treatment. No one treatment is appropriate for all people. The goal is to get people to function day to day without thinking of drugs as an option. Effective programs teach important skills for living a drug-free life. For example, people learn to handle cravings and how to avoid social situations that could lead to drug use. Another advantage of treatment is that addicted individuals and family members can achieve a healthier life by changing the patterns of behavior that trigger drug use.

The results of any program depend on the type of barbiturate, how long the drug was taken, existing medical problems, and if other drugs were used at the same time. Other issues include the time it takes to seek and get treatment and the extent of family or friend support. The Treatment Referral Helpline, at (800) 662-HELP (4357), can help teens find local treatment programs. Inpatient treatment centers usually offer four to twelve weeks of care and focus on helping teens recover from drug problems. At outpatient centers, teens participate in treatment for a few hours every day but live at home. After completing short-term programs, people may go to continuing programs for support as they adjust to living drug-free.

A group of teens shares experiences during a therapy session at a drug rehabilitation meeting. Many addicts find that both group and individual therapy are useful in their recovery and can help them lead healthy lives.

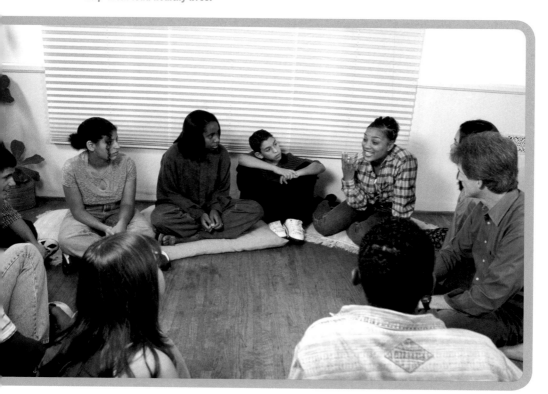

Sometimes judges will order individuals to undergo therapy. Parents, teachers, or school counselors might also recommend this route for teens. Therapists are mental health experts with specialized training and experience for assisting people with problems. Many states allow information that is discussed in therapy sessions to be confidential for people under the age of eighteen.

Teens may join support groups, which are gatherings of people who share a common problem and work together to help each other cope and recover. Support groups are the most popular type of treatment for drug addiction because they provide critical care that recovering users need to remain drug-free. Other teens are usually present during the meetings. All information is confidential and often free of charge. Recovering users frequently attend self-help group meetings several times each week. For drug addiction, they might consider Narcotics Anonymous (NA) or Rational Recovery. Teens can find local branches of these and other support groups by searching the Internet or using a telephone directory.

RECOVERY

Addicts are in recovery, but they are never cured. Recovery is a lifelong process that happens differently for each person. Experts usually recommend that teens who are recovering from addiction avoid any illegal mood-altering drugs, including alcohol, to restrain from sliding back into addiction. Many people in recovery stay drug-free the rest of their lives. Others may return to using drugs and addiction. Teens always have the choice of and chance for recovery available to them.

Prevention

Every time teens abstain from using drugs, they are promoting their own health. They send a clear message to others that they value themselves. Setting goals is a great way for people to avoid drugs and be in control of their lives. Short-term goals include finishing a homework assignment or applying for a part-time job at a local store. Other goals take longer to reach, such as learning how to play the guitar. Both types of goals are important and make it easier for teens to know what actions can interfere with reaching their goals.

A family's support can help teens develop a sense of acceptance and security and build a foundation for making decisions. Teens may want to talk about experiences at school or pressure to use drugs and how to handle that. Support from friends and peers can help teens stay away from drugs. By spending time with people who are drug-free, teens don't have to worry about being pressured to try drugs. People can join groups to meet new people and learn new skills. They can choose from a variety of groups, hobbies, sports teams, service, or special events.

A healthy lifestyle—one that holds no appeal for abusing barbiturates—requires dedication and knowledge. The results are worthwhile. Teens will have clear thinking and reasoning and a sense of being whole in mind and body.

GLOSSARY

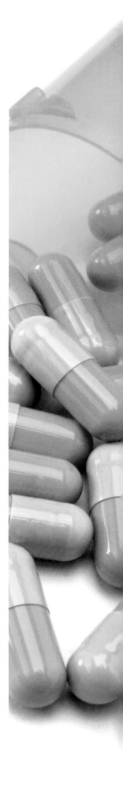

abscess An infected lesion on the skin, often found at the point where a drug user has repeatedly injected a drug into his or her body.

acquired immunodeficiency disease (AIDS) A chronic, potentially life-threatening condition caused by the human immunodeficiency virus (HIV).

addiction The compulsive feeling of need for a drug.

anesthetic A substance that brings about the loss of sensation with or without a loss of consciousness.

anxiety A condition in which real or imagined fears prevent a person from enjoying life.

barbiturate A depressant and highly addictive drug used as a sedative or anesthetic.

central nervous system (CNS) The system of the body, including the brain and spinal cord, through which sensory impulses are transmitted to control motor skills.

coma A state of profound unconsciousness that can be brought about by an overdose of barbiturates.

delirium An acute mental disturbance characterized by confused thinking and disrupted attention usually accompanied by disordered speech and hallucinations.

depressant A sedative or something that calms.

detoxification The process of freeing a drug user from a physical substance addiction.

epilepsy A medical condition causing seizures.

gangrene The complete death of skin tissue because of lack of blood flow.

human immunodeficiency virus (HIV) The virus that leads to acquired immunodeficiency disease (AIDS).

inhibition An emotion or inner instinct that tells a person to restrain his or her behavior.

insomnia The inability to sleep.

narcotic A drug that eases pain and alters the mind.

overdose A deadly, or lethal, amount of a drug that can lead to coma or death.

pharming party A party where prescription drugs are readily available in a potentially deadly mixture.

respiration The action of breathing.

sedation A state of extreme calm or fatigue that results from the use of sedative drugs, such as barbiturates.

stimulant A drug, such as caffeine or cocaine, that speeds up bodily functions and activity.

tolerance A state when the body becomes less responsive to a drug's effects because of repeated use of the drug.

withdrawal The process of discontinuing the use of a drug or other addictive substances.

FOR MORE INFORMATION

American Association of Poison Control Centers
(AAPCC)
515 King Street, Suite 510
Alexandria, VA 22314
(703) 894-1858; Help Line (800) 222-1222
Web site: http://www.aapcc.org
This organization provides a helpline for information on poisons and how to treat their
effects.

Canadian Centre on Substance Abuse (CCSA)
75 Albert Street, Suite 500
Ottawa, ON KIP 5E7
Canada
(613) 235-4048
Web site: http://www.ccsa.ca
The Canadian Centre on Substance Abuse provides leadership and research for national
programs to reduce drug-related harm.

Center for Substance Abuse Treatment
5600 Fishers Lane Rockwall II
Rockville, MD 20857
(301) 443-0365
Web site: http://prevention.samhsa.gov
The center, which is part of the U.S. Department

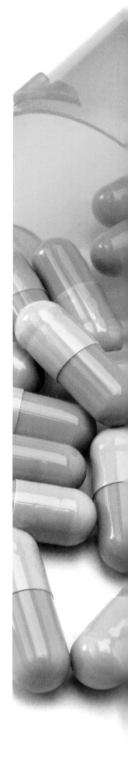

of Health and Human Services, promotes the quality and availability of community-based substance abuse treatment services for individuals and families who need them.

Narcotics Anonymous (NA)
P.O. Box 9999
Van Nuys, CA 91409
(818) 773-9999
Web site: http://www.na.org
Narcotics Anonymous offers recovery from the effects of addiction through a twelve-step program, including regular attendance at group meetings.

National Council on Alcoholism and Drug Dependence (NCADD)
217 Broadway, Suite 712
New York, NY 10007
(212) 269-7797
Web site: http://www.ncadd.org
NCADD provides information on drug abuse prevention, where to find treatment, and where recovery support groups are located.

National Institute on Drug Abuse (NIDA)
6001 Executive Boulevard, Room 5213
Bethesda, MD 20892-9561
(301) 443-1124

Web site: http://www.nida.nih.gov

This federal agency brings the power of scientific research to bear on the problems of drug abuse and addiction. The Web site offers a wealth of information about prescription drugs and other drugs that are abused.

The Partnership at Drugfree.org

352 Park Avenue South, 9th Floor

New York, NY 10010

(212) 922-1560

Web site: http://www.drugfree.org

The Partnership at Drugfree.org is a drug abuse prevention, intervention, treatment, and recovery resource. It especially provides information and assistance about teen drug abuse and addiction for families.

Web Sites

Due to the changing nature of Internet links, Rosen Publishing has developed an online list of Web sites related to the subject of this book. This site is updated regularly. Please use this link to access the list:

http://www.rosenlinks.com/DAC/Barb

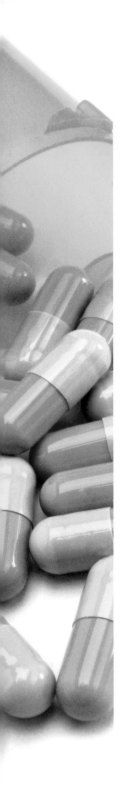

FOR FURTHER READING

Abadinsky, Howard. *Drug Use and Abuse.* Independence, KY: Wadsworth Publishing, 2013.

Adamec, Christine. *Barbiturates and Other Depressants.* New York, NY: Chelsea House Publishers, 2011.

Bandry, Yvette L. *Help for Drug Addicts: A Self-Help Book About Drug Addiction Symptoms, Drug Abuse Intervention, Drug Rehab, the 12-Step Program and Other Treatments So You Can Heal Yourself from Substance Abuse.* Charleston, SC: CreateSpace Publishing, 2011.

Bjornlund, Lydia. *Prescription Drugs.* San Diego, CA: ReferencePoint Press, 2009.

DeHaven, Bradley V. *How to Prevent, Detect, Treat and Live with the Addict Among Us.* Charleston, SC: CreateSpace Publishing, 2012.

Engdahl, Sylvia. *Prescription Drugs* (Current Controversies). Detroit, MI: Greenhaven Press/ Gale Cengage Learning, 2008.

Francis, K. A. *Drugs.* North Mankato, MN: Cherry Lake Publishers, 2009.

Haley, John. *The Truth About Drugs.* New York, NY: Facts On File, 2009.

Jensen, Taylor S. *Understanding Drugs and Drug Addiction: Treatment to Recovery and Real*

Accounts of Ex-Addicts. Charleston, SC: CreateSpace Publishing, 2012.

Klosterman, Lorrie. *The Facts About Depressants.* Salt Lake City, UT: Benchmark Books, 2009.

Kuhar, Michael. *The Addicted Brain: Why We Abuse Drugs, Alcohol, and Nicotine.* Upper Saddle River, NJ: FT Press, 2011.

Leonard, Basia, and Jeremy Roberts. *The Truth About Prescription Drugs.* New York, NY: Rosen Publishing, 2012.

Mather, Linda. *I Shall Be Clean: Self-Help Book for Addiction.* Charleston, SC: CreateSpace, 2012.

Medina, Sarah. *Know the Facts: Drugs.* New York, NY: Rosen Publishing, 2009.

Nelson, Blake. *Recovery Road.* New York, NY: Scholastic Press, 2011.

Nelson, David. *Teen Drug Abuse.* Detroit, MI: Greenhaven Press, 2010.

Pampel, Fred. *Prescription Drugs.* New York, NY: Facts On File, 2010.

Porterfield, Jason. *Downers: Depressant Abuse.* New York, NY: Rosen Publishing, 2008.

Simmons, Linda L. *The Everything Health Guide to Addiction and Recovery: Control Your Behavior and Build a Better Life.* Avon, MA: Adams Media, 2008.

Wolny, Philip. *Abusing Prescription Drugs.* New York, NY: Rosen Publishing, 2008.

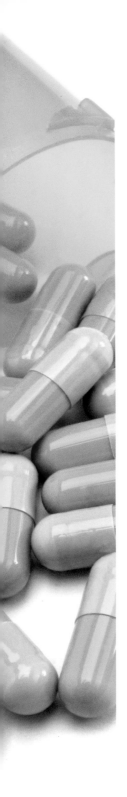

BIBLIOGRAPHY

Barry, J. Dave, and Christopher Beach. "Barbiturate Abuse." 2013. Retrieved January 29, 2013 (http://www.webmd.com/mental-health/barbiturate-abuse).

Converse, Beverly. *Everything Changes: Help for Families of Newly Recovering Addicts.* Center City, MN: Hazelden, 2009.

Ellis, Ross. "Teen 'Pharm' or 'Pharming' Parties—AKA 'Punch Bowl Parties.'" March 3, 2010. Retrieved January 4, 2013 (http://www.examiner.com/article/teen-pharm-or-pharming-parties-aka-punch-bowl-parties).

Erowid. "Drug Testing Basics." September 27, 2010. Retrieved January 3, 2013 (http://www.erowid.org/psychoactives/testing/testing_info1.shtm).

Lameman, Beth Aileen. "Effects of Substance Abuse on Families." 2013. Retrieved January 29, 2013 (http://www.chicagotribune.com/sns-health-addiction-families,0,2311189.story).

MedlinePlus. "Prescription Drug Abuse." August 30, 2012. Retrieved December 29, 2012 (http://www.nlm.nih.gov/medlineplus/prescriptiondrugabuse.html).

Parker, Jim. "Barbiturates: Show Stoppers." 2007. Retrieved January 3, 2013 (http://www.doitnow.org/pages/111.html).

Recovery Connection. "Drug Addiction Treatment." 2013. Retrieved January 2, 2013 (http://www.recoveryconnection .org/drug-addiction-treatment).

U.S. Drug Enforcement Agency. "Barbiturates." 2012. Retrieved December 28, 2012 (http://www.justthinktwice.com/drugs/ barbiturates.html).

U.S. National Institute on Drug Abuse. "Diagnosis and Treatment of Drug Abuse in Family Practice." 2006. Retrieved January 25, 2013 (http://archives.drugabuse.gov/diagnosis-treatment/ diagnosis1.html).

U.S. National Institute on Drug Abuse. "Monitoring the Future Data Tables and Figures." December 2012. Retrieved January 2, 2013 (http://www.monitoringthefuture.org/data/12data/ pr12t2.pdf).

U.S. National Institute on Drug Abuse. "Prescription Drugs." February 19, 2013. Retrieved February 20, 2013 (http://teens .drugabuse.gov/drug-facts/prescription-drugs).

U.S. National Institute on Drug Abuse. "Prescription Use and Abuse." October 2011. Retrieved December 27, 2012 (http://www.drugabuse.gov/publications/research-reports/ prescription-drugs).

U.S. Substance Abuse and Mental Health Services Administration. "Results from the 2011 National Survey on Drug Use and Health: Summary of National Findings and Detailed Tables." December 11, 2012. Retrieved December 15, 2012 (http://www.samhsa.gov/data/ NSDUH/2011SummNatFindDetTables).

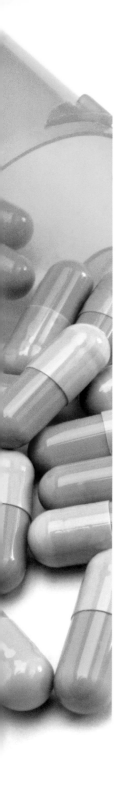

INDEX

About the Author

Judy Monroe Peterson has earned two master's degrees and is the author of more than sixty educational books for young people, including books on the dangers of antidepressants, herbal drugs, steroids, nicotine, and alcohol. She is a former health care, technical, and academic librarian and college faculty member; a biologist and research scientist; and curriculum editor with more than thirty years of experience. Currently, she is a writer and editor of K–12 and post–high school curriculum materials on a variety of subjects, including biology, life science, and the environment.

Photo Credits

Cover, p. 1 serav/Shutterstock.com; pp. 4–5 Diana Taliun/Shutterstock.com; pp. 8, 18, 28, 36, 45, 53, 55, 58, 60, 62 Charles Shapiro/Shutterstock.com; p. 9 Apic/Hulton Archive/Getty Images; p. 11 Science Source; p. 14 Zoonar/Thinkstock; p. 19 Digital Vision/Thinkstock; p. 21 Juanmonino/the Agency Collection/Getty Images; pp. 24, 26, 40, 43 © AP Images; p. 30 Image Source/Getty Images; p. 32 SnowWhiteImages/Shutterstock.com; p. 33 David Parker/Science Photo Library/Getty Images; p. 37 Paul Bradbury/Caiaimage/Getty Images; p. 46 Huy Lam/First Light/Getty Images; p. 50 © Mary Kate Denny/PhotoEdit.

Designer: Sam Zavieh; Editor: Kathy Kuhtz Campbell; Photo Researcher: Karen Huang